Journeying Jiao

Intentionally make happen

Created by Luke Thompson

Co-author Caroline Bennett

Illustrated by Kat Willott

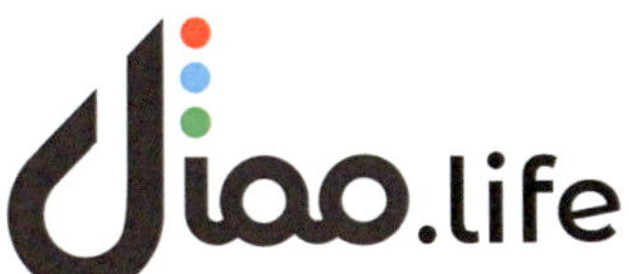

Published by Jiao Ltd
Jiao.life

Scan the QR codes to access the digital book or listen to the audio book.

Audiobook

Digital Book

The Seven Stages of Switch Development

Journeying Jiao is part of the Switch Heroes, social stories created to support switch-users with their Switch progression. The Switch Heroes series is part of the Seven Stages of Switch Development, created by Occupational Therapist and AT specialist Luke Thompson.

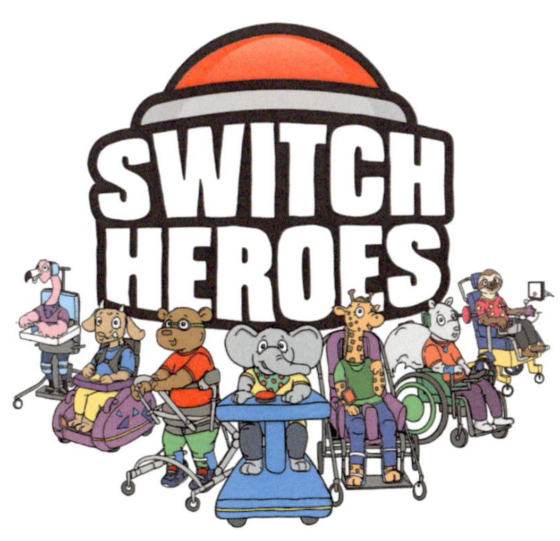

Jiao is on a Journey

She's going to come and play

She has got something special

That she wants to say

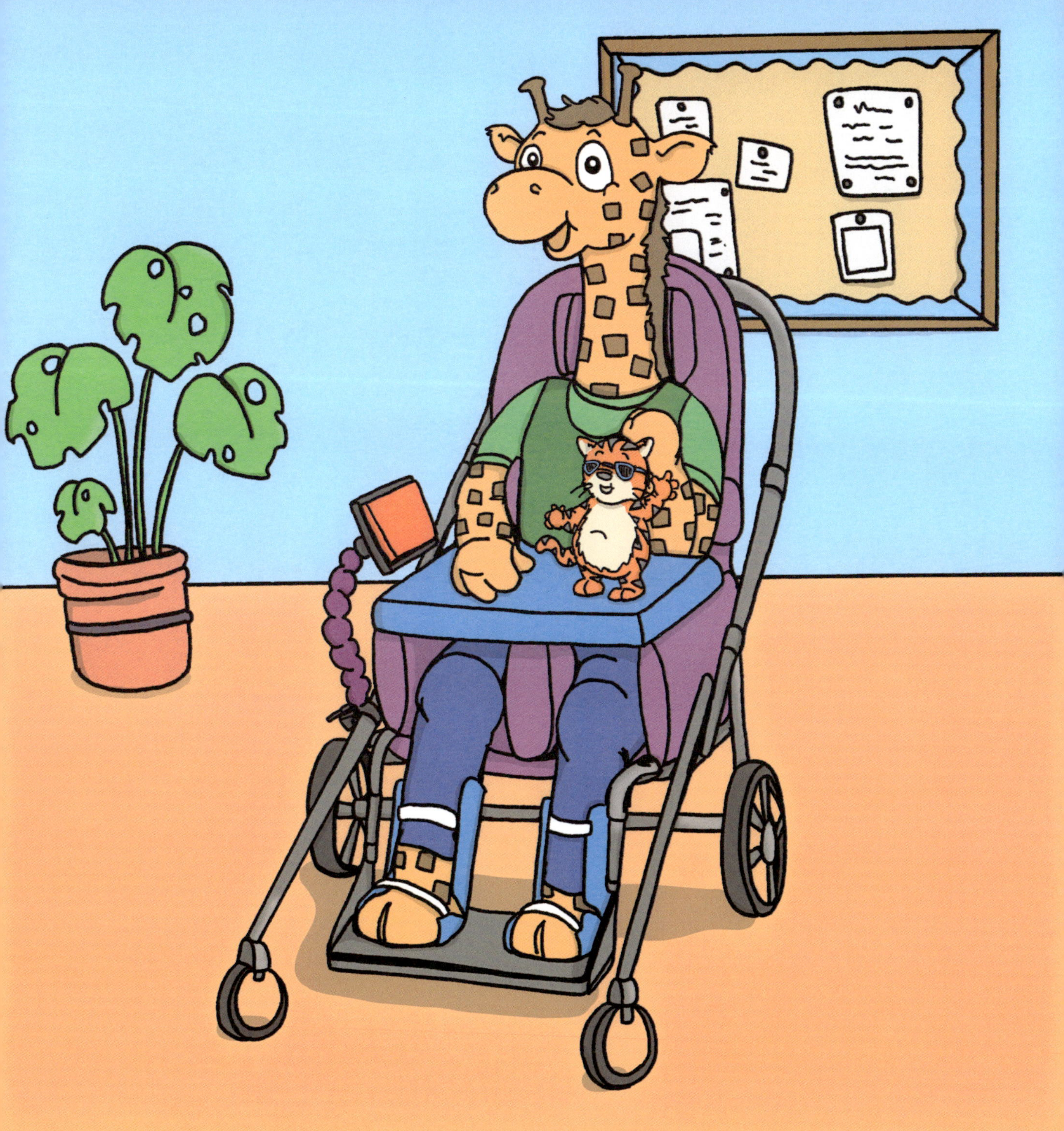

“Have you got your switch?

“Your big orange square?”

“Have you got your
switch positioned

Properly on your chair?”

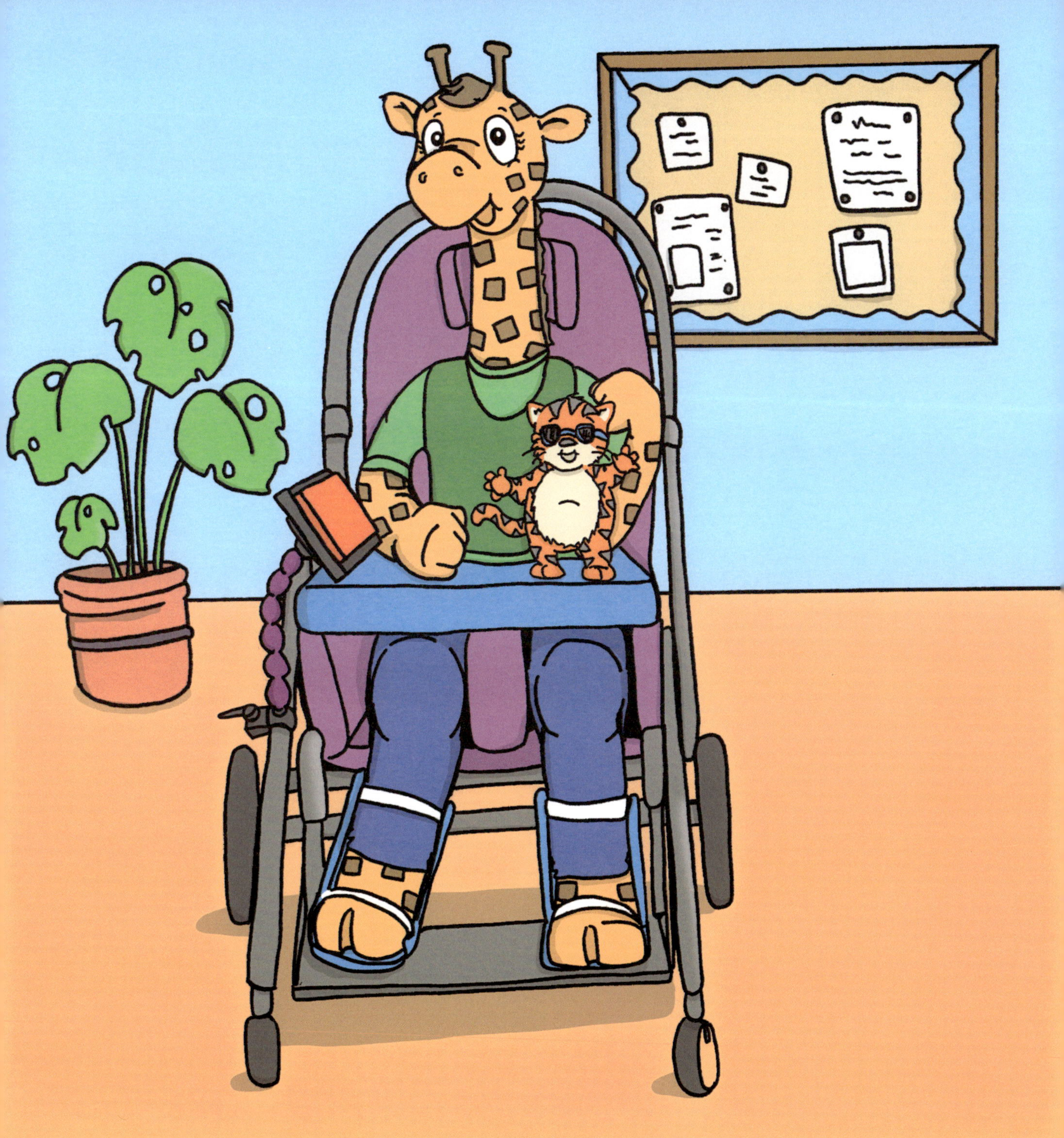

Jiao’s got a clever toy
And when she presses
And holds her switch
It dances!
What a joy

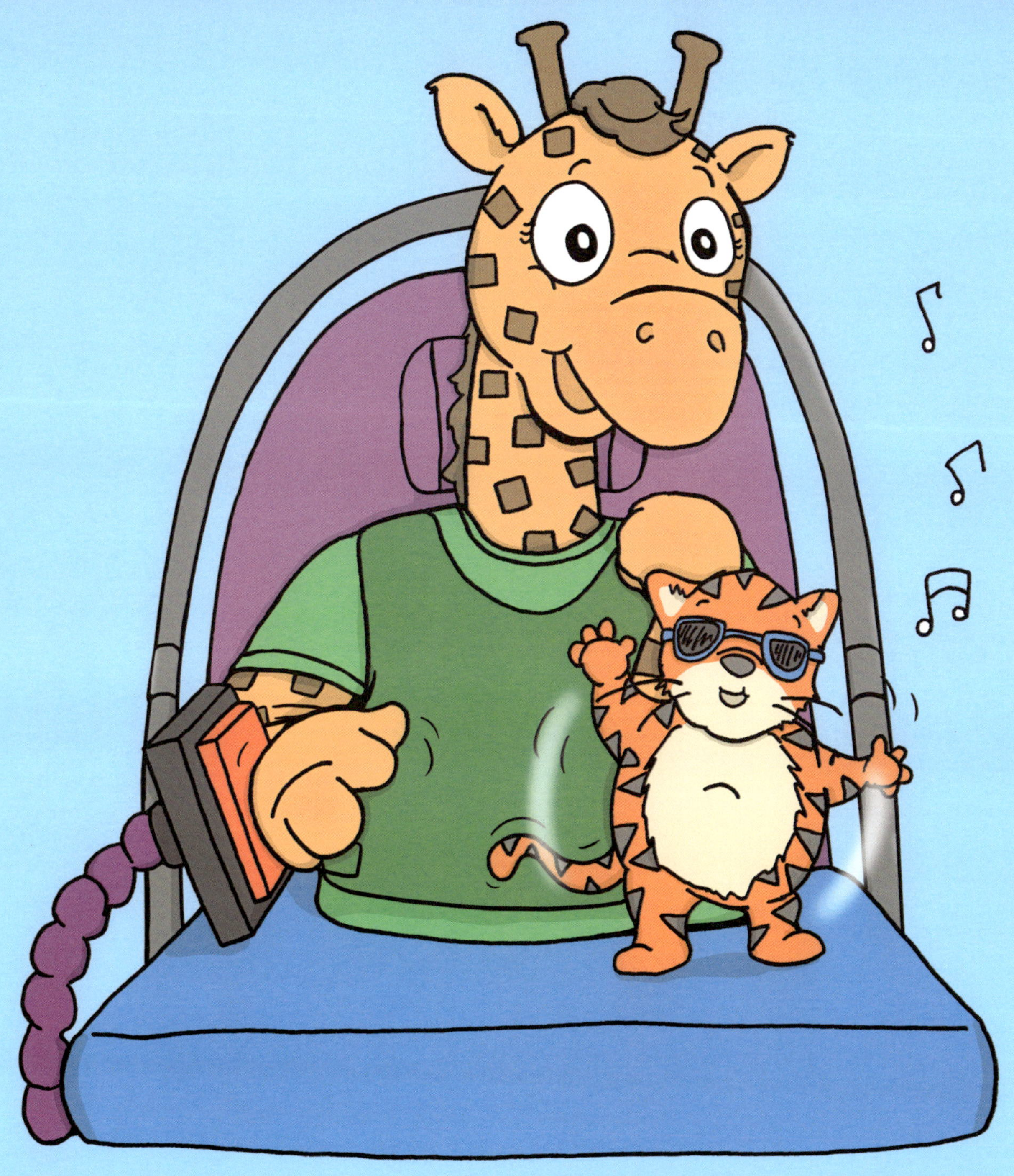

Can you press and
hold your switch?

One, two, three

What dancing, singing, joyful fun

For you, Jiao, and me

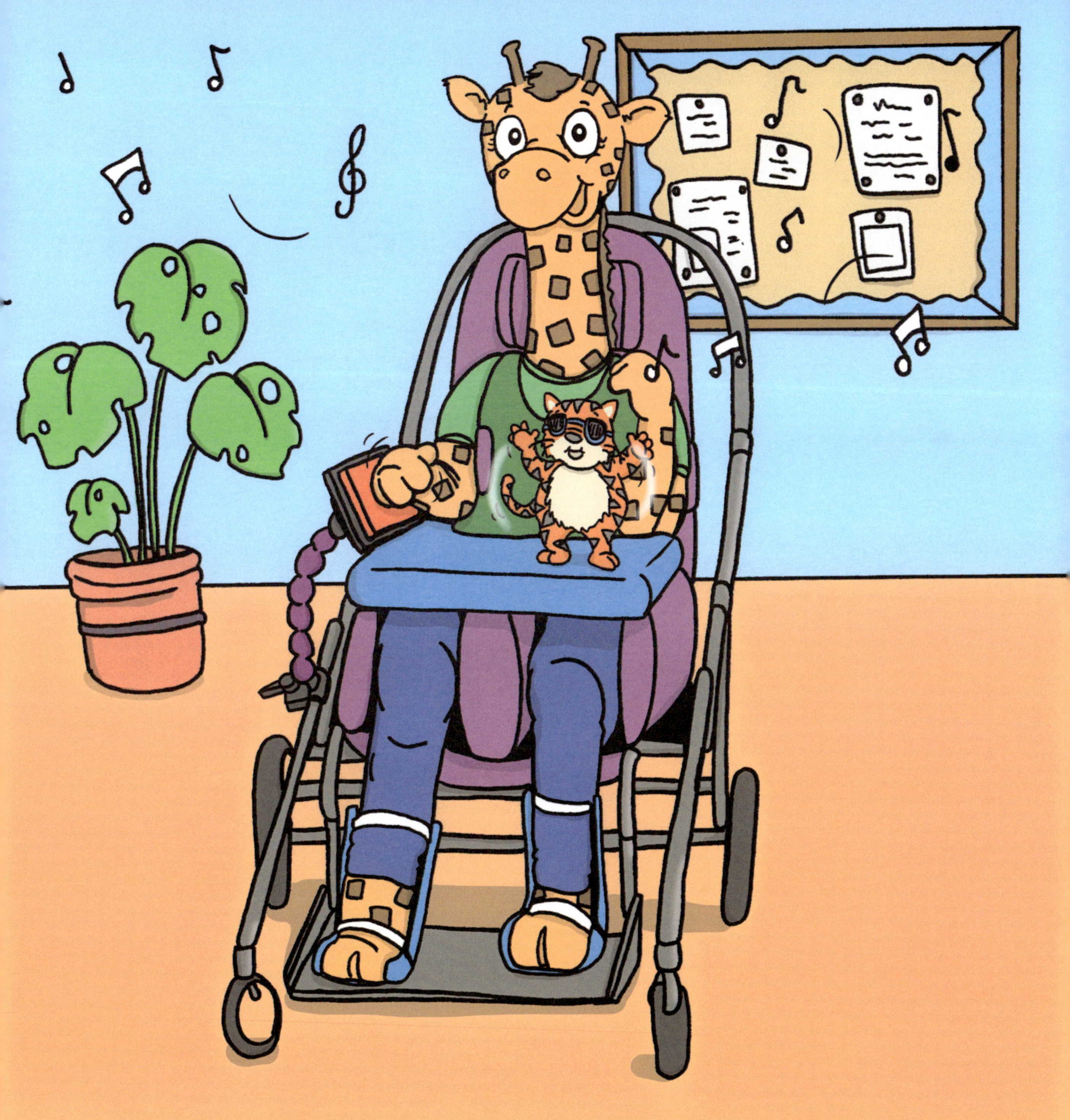

When you push and hold your
switch, the fan can blow your hair

When you push and hold your
switch, you can spin in your chair

When you push and hold your
switch, you can play a song

Can you push and hold
your switch? – you can,
but for how long?’

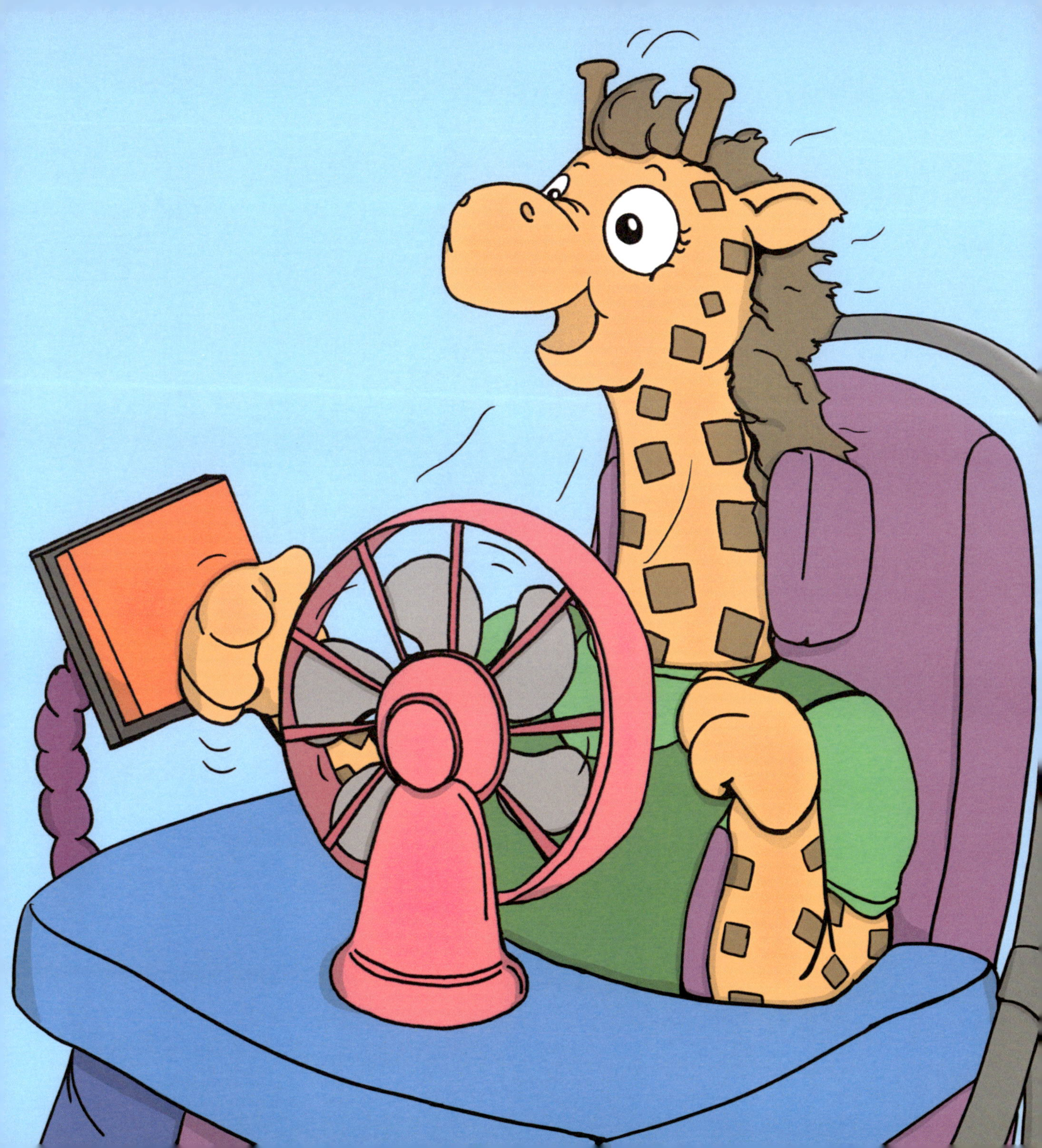

Thank you, Jiao it's been fun
We've learned something new
When we want things to happen
We know just what to do

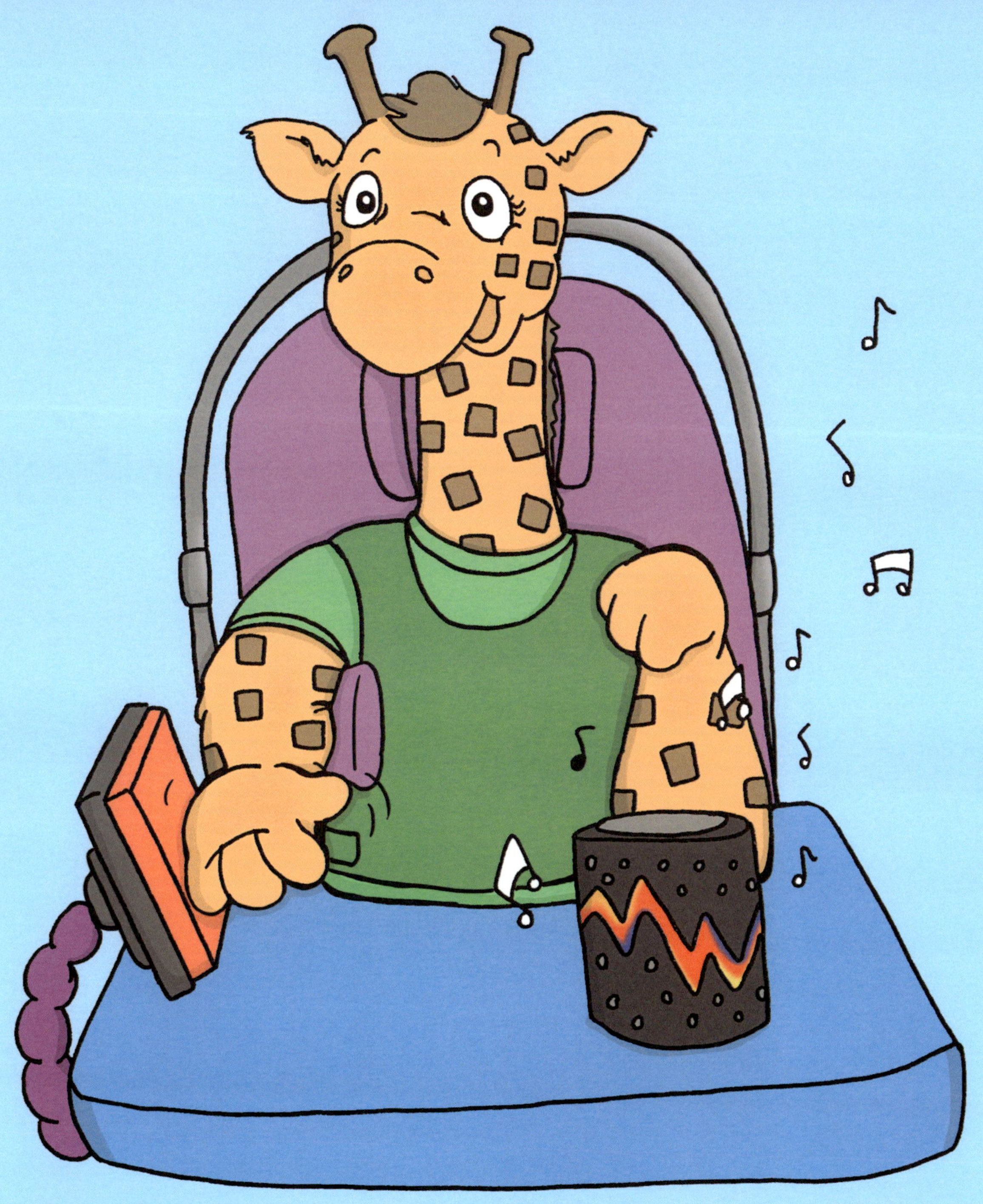

We focus, push and
hold our switch

When we want to play

Then we can start to
use our switch

All throughout the day

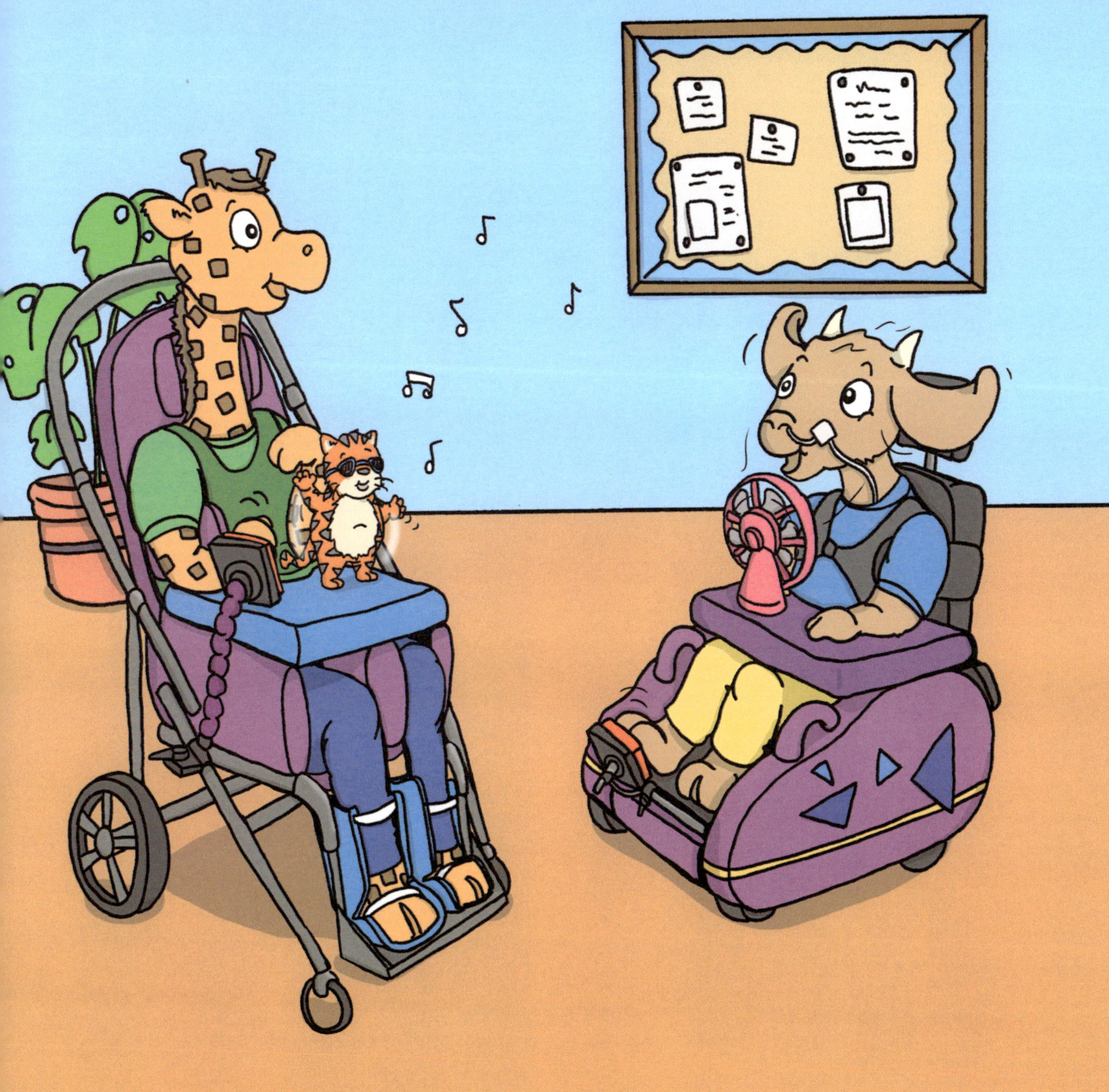

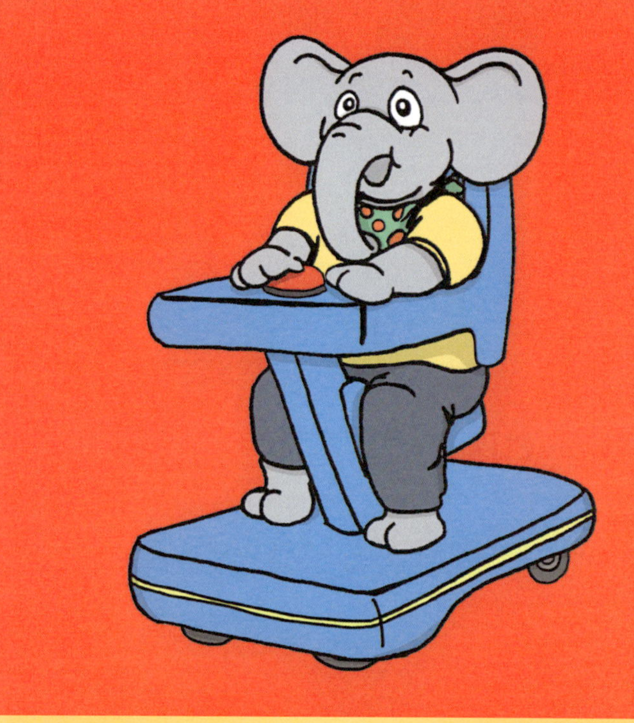
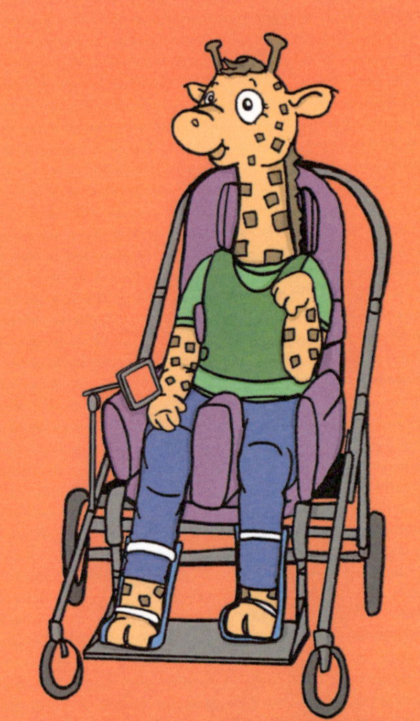
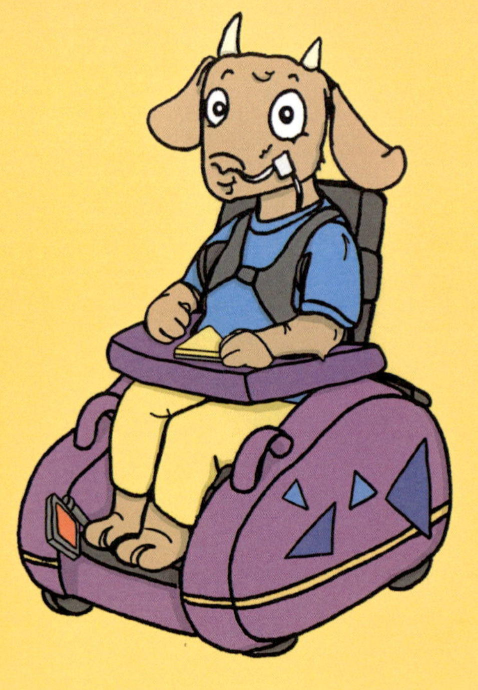
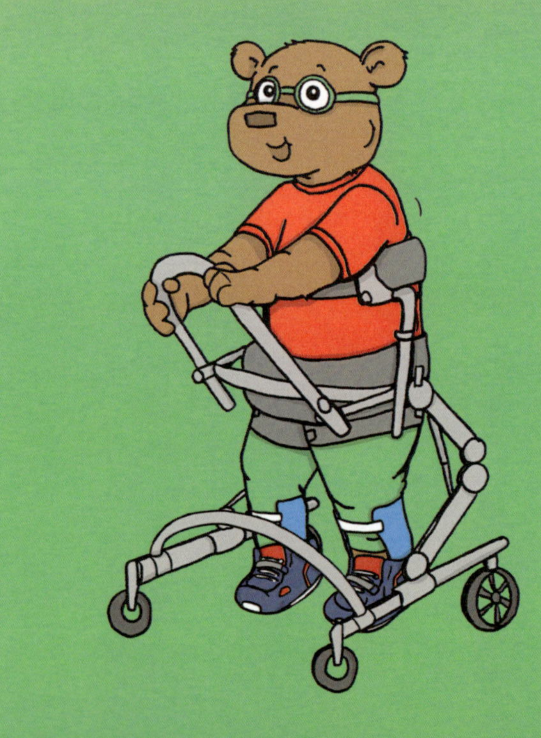

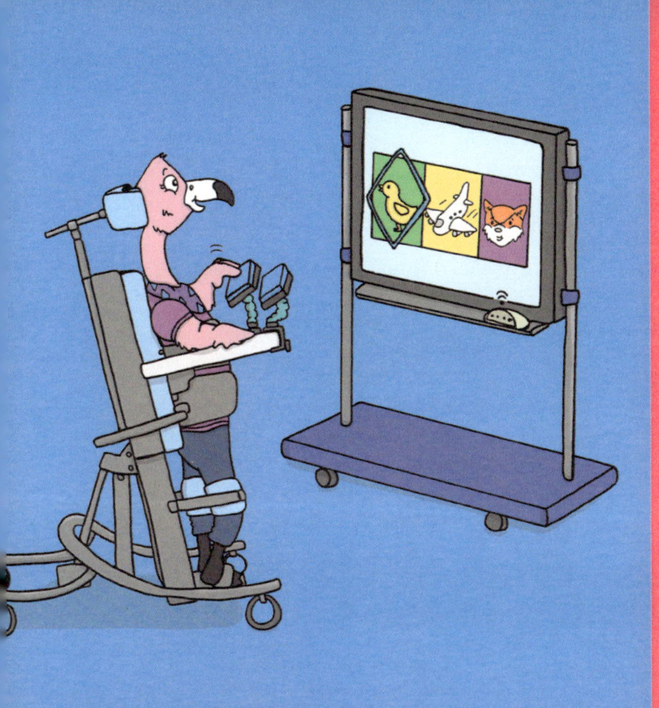

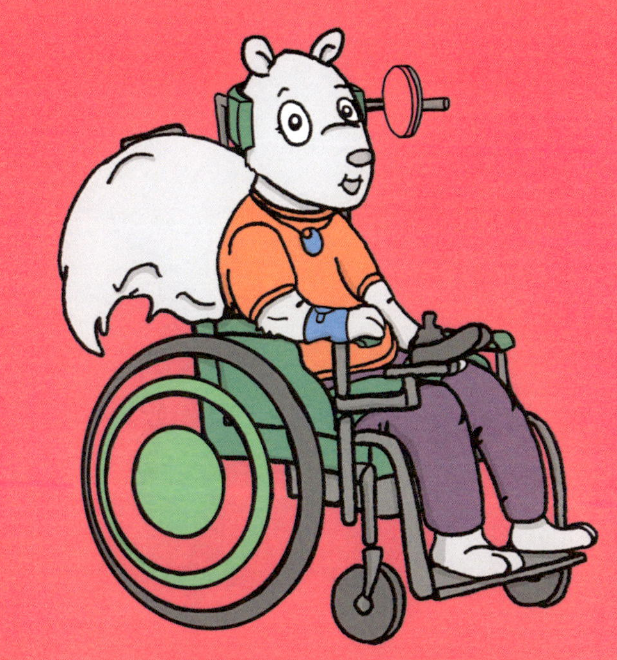

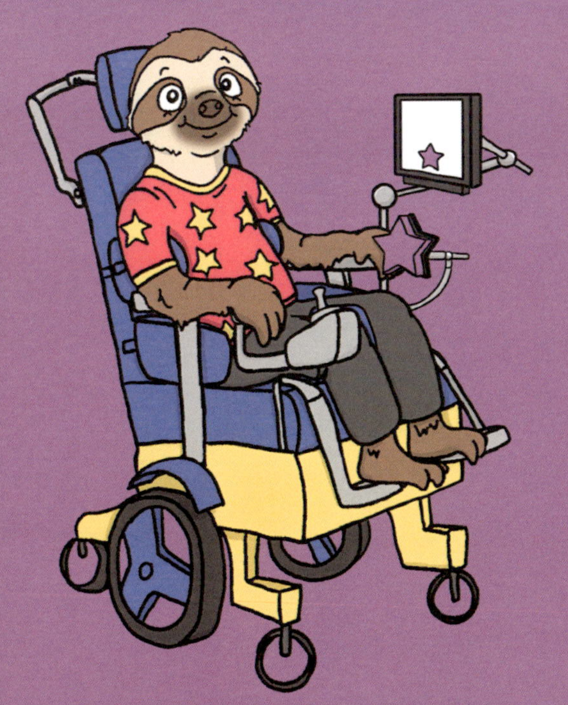

Photo of you!

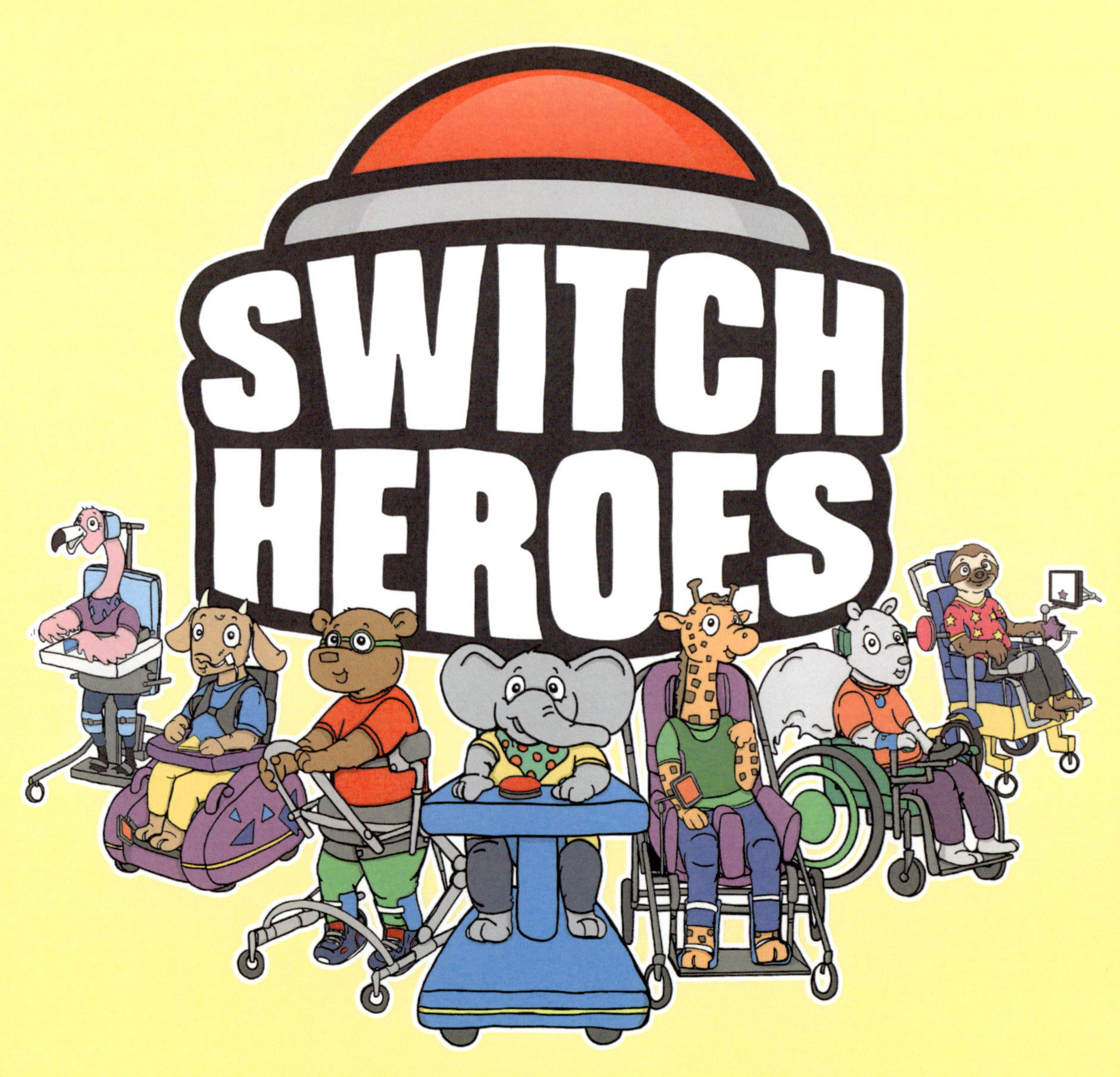
SWITCH
HEROES

The Seven Stages of Switch Development

The Seven Stages of Switch Development is a resource designed for switch-users, their families, caregivers and those who assist them in using switches. It features child-friendly characters and stories that support everyones learning.

The framework provides a helpful reference for measuring and tracking progress while offering flexibility to accommodate the unique needs and preferences of each switch-user.

Written directly to the switch-user, the framework can be read to them if they are unable to read it themselves. Our aim is to ensure that those supporting the child/switch-user can prioritise the child's needs and perspective in the process of developing their switch skills. We have seen the impact of involving the child in the learning process. Seeking their input and feedback regularly empowers them to take an active role in their development and combat learned helplessness.

Adapted from: Bean, I. (2011). Switch Progression Learning Journeys Road Map. Inclusive Technology.
Burkhart, L. (2018). Stepping Stones to Switch Access. Perspectives of the ASHA Special Interest Groups, 3(12), pp.33-44. doi:https://doi/10.1044/persp3.sig12.33.

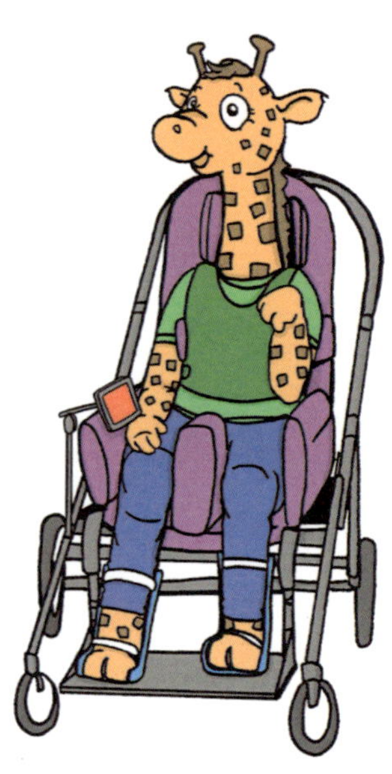

Stage 2
Intentionally make happen
Journeying Jiao the Giraffe
Square/Orange

Definition

Journeying Jiao is the stage where you start to intentionally make something happen when using switches. You will increasingly understand that when you press - or press and hold - a switch, it causes the activity/effect to happen. Through lots of repetition, you will also start to develop the motor skills to press the switch with your body.

This stage has two steps, the knowing (cognitive) step and the doing, motor skill (physical/body movement) step. It is important to first focus on the knowing step. Activities need to be fun and of interest to you, with the switch being placed where you can most easily reach it.

The knowing step is when you start to show anticipation and understanding about the switch activities. Moving the switch to different locations for you to use different parts of your body helps you to know that wherever the switch is, when you press it, the activities are still activated. Moving a single switch also prepares you for the next stage (playing with two switches) and provides you with more options for using switches in the future. For example, if you get tired or hurt from using one switch site you can change to another.

Now that you know more about what the switch does, you need to practice repeating the body movement until it becomes automatic. This happens when you succeed and have the desire to keep using your switch. It is a good idea to have a main and backup switch location, but it is also important to try out other options regularly. At this stage, the switch activity should now be completely abstract from the switch.

Milestones

- Anticipating cause and effect: You will understand that pressing the switch causes a specific activity/effect to happen
- Developing motor skills: You will have developed the motor skills necessary to intentionally press the switch with your preferred body part
- Moving the switch: You will have experience of the switch being moved and activated by multiple body parts. This helps you to understand that regardless of the location, the switch still activates activities. This will prepare you for the next stage (using a second switch)
- Abstract switch activities: You will know that the switch can cause something to happen that may not be directly related to it – a toy moving on a table away from the switch
- Increase in time: You will be able to engage in motivating switch activities for longer periods of time

Top tips

- Provide ample opportunities for the switch-user to use switches throughout the day. Frequent repetition will develop motor skills and automaticity
- To keep the switch-user motivated, use a variety of switch activities that are of interest to them
- Experiment with different switch locations and body parts for activation
- Avoid saying the phrase, ‘press the switch’. Instead, give them verbal encouragement related to the activity (e.g. ‘can you turn the light on?’ or ‘let’s make the toy move/dance/sing!’)
- Optimise the environment to support the child’s success with the switch, including positioning the switch at an accessible height/distance and minimising distractions. Regularly assess and adjust the environment as needed to support progress
- Consider the child’s sensory and regulation needs and provide appropriate supports
- Focus on building the child’s understanding and ability to intentionally press the switch rather than just focusing on how they press it
- Identify and provide a primary and secondary switch site, but also encourage exploration of alternative options

Activities

- Use a range of switch-adapted toys
- Use a switch interface that connects and controls mains powered household appliances, such as a mixer, hair dryer, or sensory lights
- Use a voice-output switch to record a range of motivating commands, such as 'Tickle me, Mummy!' or 'More bubbles!'
- Use a voice-output switch to take part in a story, adding a recording such as, 'turn the page' or say a repeated line of the story
- Computer games: For example, games that require the child to press a switch to make things happen, such as cause and effect or simple story games. Create a gameplay on Tar Heel Gameplay to allow the switch-user to continue playing their favourite YouTube video
- Sensory activities: Activities that allow the child to control sensory stimulation by pressing the switch, such as bubble machines, vibrating pillows, or sensory balls

Instead of a prompt hierarchy where the type of prompt increase in support level, we recommend our one prompt switch support cycle. Find out more at Jiao.life

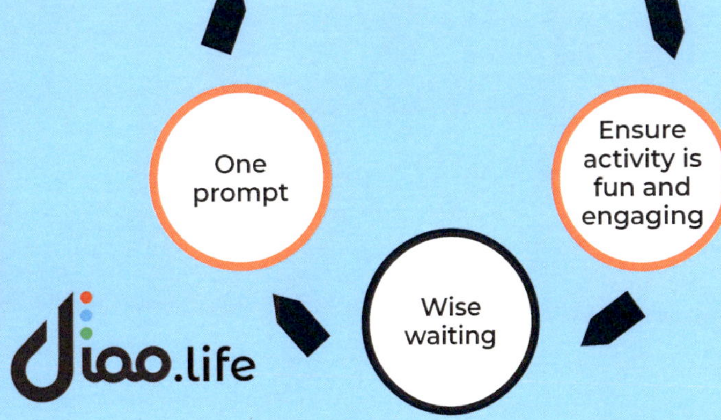

The Assessment Tool

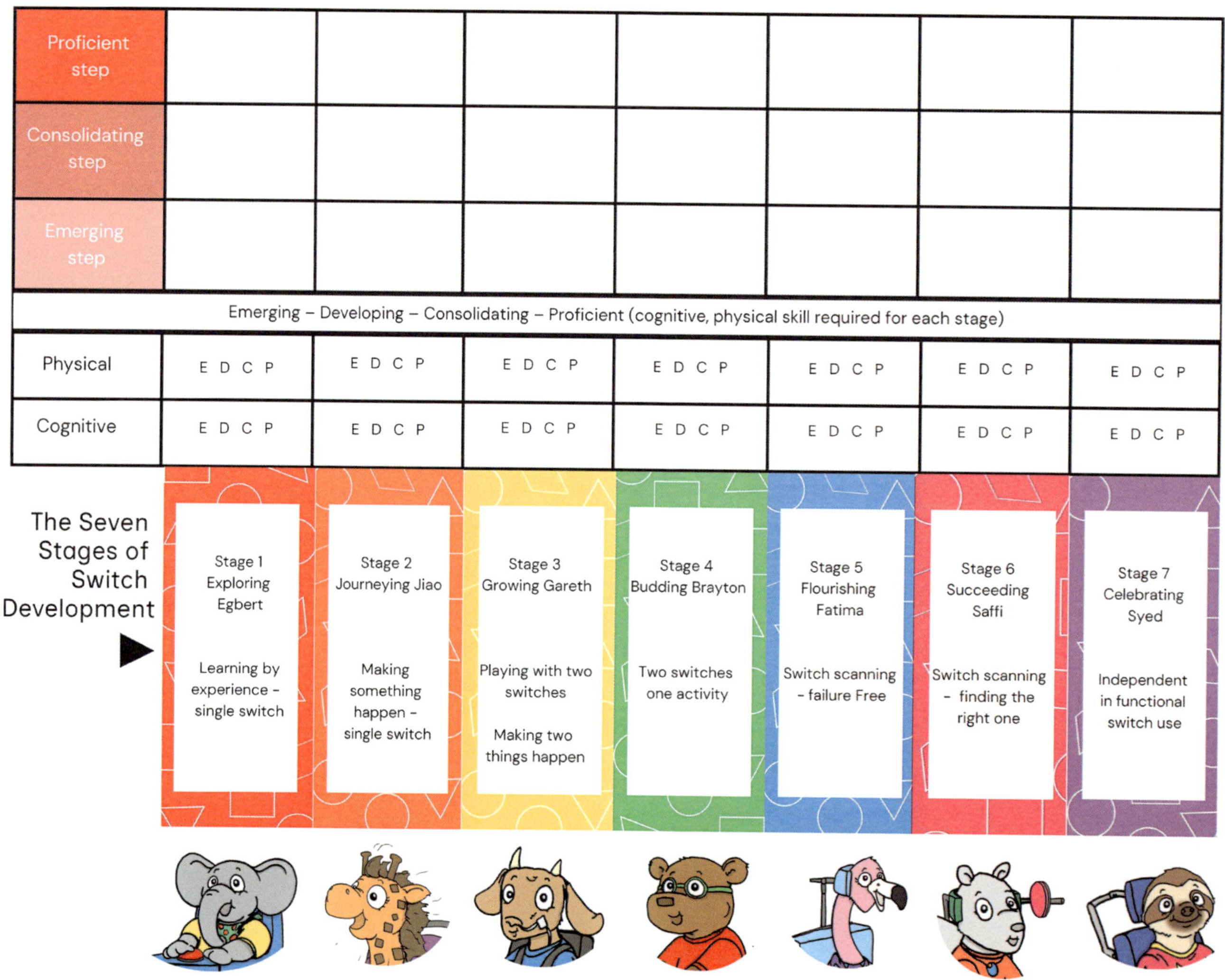

Proficient step							
Consolidating step							
Emerging step							
Emerging – Developing – Consolidating – Proficient (cognitive, physical skill required for each stage)							
Physical	E D C P	E D C P	E D C P	E D C P	E D C P	E D C P	E D C P
Cognitive	E D C P	E D C P	E D C P	E D C P	E D C P	E D C P	E D C P
The Seven Stages of Switch Development ▶	Stage 1 Exploring Egbert Learning by experience - single switch	Stage 2 Journeying Jiao Making something happen - single switch	Stage 3 Growing Gareth Playing with two switches Making two things happen	Stage 4 Budding Brayton Two switches one activity	Stage 5 Flourishing Fatima Switch scanning - failure Free	Stage 6 Succeeding Saffi Switch scanning - finding the right one	Stage 7 Celebrating Syed Independent in functional switch use

Print version available at jiao.life

How to use the assessment tool

- The stages of switch development are not mutually exclusive, so progress can be made across multiple stages simultaneously
- Once a step is completed, mark it off and add the date
- The assessment tool can be used for goal setting, where helpers can add target dates and change the text/box colour accordingly
- There is a stream for assessing cognitive and physical skill development, divided into four steps for each stage (Emerging, Developing, Consolidating and Proficient)
- Helpers should consider the cognitive and physical skills required for each level
- This additional stream can help identify areas that may require additional support and highlight strengths and weaknesses for targeted interventions

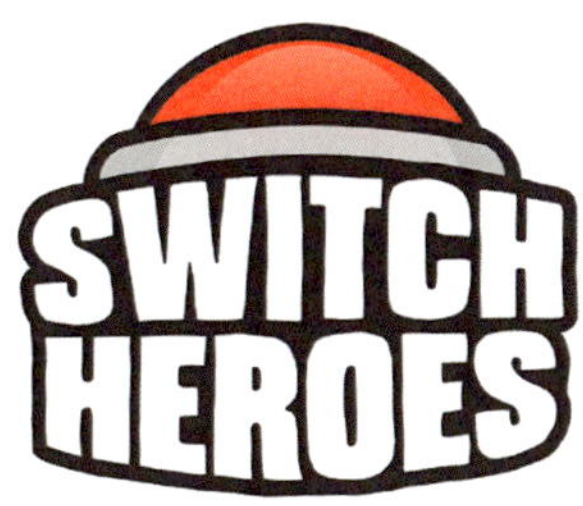

At Jiao Ltd, we are dedicated to empowering individuals through innovative assistive technology solutions.

We provide personalised services and training to help children, families, and professionals navigate the world of assistive tech. For more resources, training options, or to learn how we can support you, visit Jiao.life or get in touch with us directly. We look forward to hearing from you!

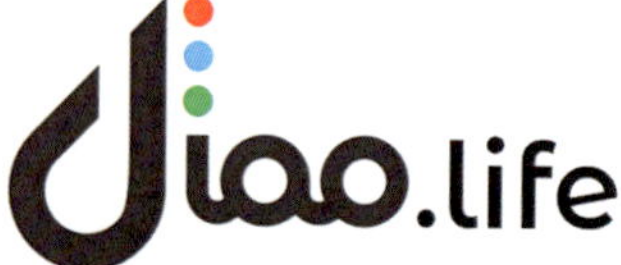

This is to certify that

____

is intentionally making things happen

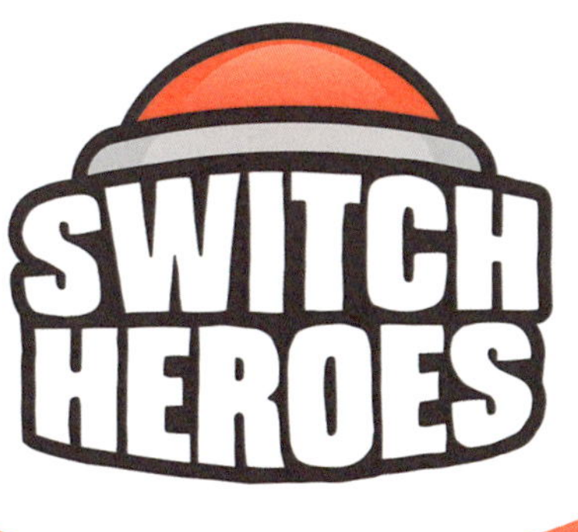

Notes

www.ingramcontent.com/pod-product-compliance
Ingram Content Group UK Ltd.
Pitfield, Milton Keynes, MK11 3LW, UK
UKRC032027290726
14090UKWH00008B/483

* 9 7 8 1 8 0 3 2 9 9 7 4 7 *